This publication is intended to provide educational information for the reader on the covered subjects. It is not intended to take the place of personalized medical counseling, diagnosis, and treatment from a trained healthcare professional.

ISBN 978-1-998740-01-7 (Paperback)
ISBN 978-1-998740-02-4 (eBook)

Printed and bound in USA
Published by Loons Press

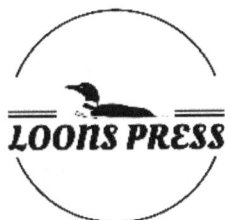

I0106285

LOONS PRESS

Table Of Contents

How To Prevent Glaucoma

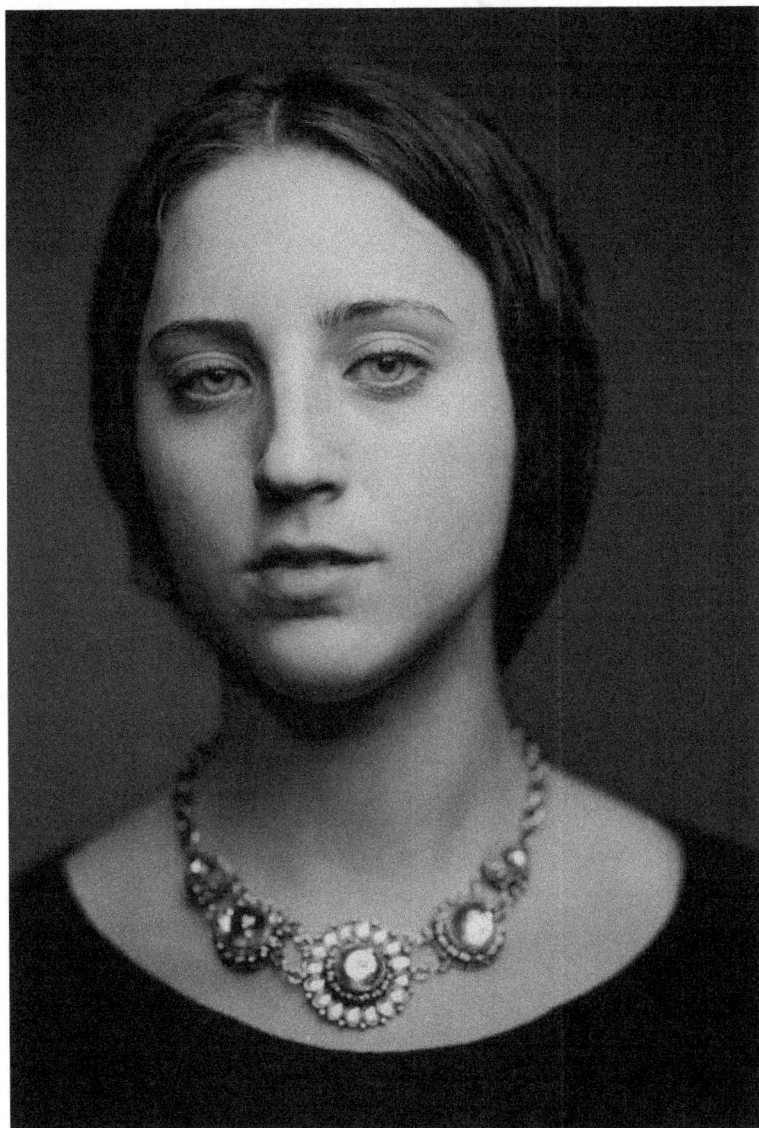

Your Action Plan for Healthy Eyes

Chapter 1
Understanding Glaucoma

What is Glaucoma?

Glaucoma is a group of eye diseases that can lead to progressive damage to the optic nerve, often resulting in vision loss and potentially blindness.

This condition is typically associated with increased intraocular pressure (IOP), which can occur when the fluid in the eye does not drain properly. The optic nerve is crucial for transferring visual information from the eye to the brain, and any damage to it can severely impact one's sight.

Understanding glaucoma is essential for anyone concerned about their eye health, as early detection and management can significantly reduce the risk of severe outcomes.

There are several types of glaucoma, the most common being open-angle glaucoma and angle-closure glaucoma. Open-angle glaucoma is characterized by a gradual increase in eye pressure and often occurs without noticeable symptoms in its early stages. This can lead individuals to be unaware of their condition until significant damage has occurred.

On the other hand, angle-closure glaucoma is less common but can present suddenly with intense symptoms such as severe eye pain, nausea, and blurred vision. Recognizing the differences between these types is crucial for understanding how to prevent and manage the disease.

Risk factors for developing glaucoma include age, family history, ethnic background, and certain medical conditions such as diabetes or hypertension. Individuals over the age of 60 are at a higher risk, and African Americans are particularly susceptible to developing glaucoma at an earlier age and with more severe consequences.

Regular eye examinations are vital for early detection, especially for those with known risk factors. Eye care professionals can monitor eye pressure and assess the optic nerve for any signs of damage during these check-ups.

Preventive measures play a significant role in managing eye health and reducing the risk of glaucoma. Maintaining a healthy lifestyle, including regular exercise, a balanced diet rich in leafy greens and omega-3 fatty acids, and avoiding smoking, can contribute to overall eye health.

Additionally, staying hydrated and managing other health conditions, such as diabetes and hypertension, can help lower the risk of developing glaucoma. It is also advisable to be aware of any changes in vision and seek immediate medical attention if any concerning symptoms arise.

In conclusion, understanding what glaucoma is and how it can affect vision is essential for individuals concerned about their eye health. By recognizing the types of glaucoma, identifying risk factors, and implementing preventive measures, one can take proactive steps in safeguarding their eyesight. Regular eye exams and awareness of personal health can lead to timely interventions, ultimately preserving vision and enhancing overall quality of life.

Types of Glaucoma

Glaucoma is a group of eye conditions that damage the optic nerve, often associated with increased intraocular pressure. Understanding the various types of glaucoma is crucial for early detection and effective management. The two primary categories of glaucoma are open-angle and angle-closure glaucoma, each with unique characteristics, symptoms, and treatment approaches.

Open-angle glaucoma, the most common form, develops gradually and often goes unnoticed until significant vision loss occurs. This type is characterized by a slow blockage of the drainage canals in the eye, leading to a gradual build-up of pressure.

Closed-angle glaucoma, also known as angle-closure glaucoma, occurs when the drainage angle of the eye becomes blocked, causing a rapid increase in intraocular pressure. This type can present with sudden and severe symptoms, including intense eye pain, headache, nausea, vomiting, and blurred vision.

It is considered a medical emergency, requiring immediate treatment to prevent permanent vision loss. Recognizing the symptoms of closed-angle glaucoma is vital, as timely intervention can save vision.

Another important subtype is normal-tension glaucoma, where optic nerve damage occurs despite normal eye pressure levels. The exact cause of this condition remains unclear, but it may be related to poor blood flow to the optic nerve or other factors influencing nerve health. Individuals with a family history of glaucoma or those who have certain medical conditions may be at higher risk for normal-tension glaucoma, making regular eye exams essential for early detection.

Secondary glaucoma, which can arise from other medical conditions or injuries to the eye, deserves attention as well. This type can result from inflammatory diseases, trauma, or complications from other eye surgeries.

Identifying the underlying cause is crucial for effective treatment and management. Patients with secondary glaucoma may exhibit symptoms similar to other types, emphasizing the importance of comprehensive eye examinations.

Finally, congenital glaucoma occurs in infants and young children due to abnormal development of the eye's drainage system. Early signs can include excessive tearing, sensitivity to light, and an enlarged eye. Timely diagnosis and treatment are critical for preserving vision in children with congenital glaucoma.

Understanding these different types of glaucoma empowers individuals to seek appropriate care and take preventive measures to protect their eye health. Regular eye exams, awareness of risk factors, and prompt attention to any concerning symptoms are essential components of a proactive approach to preventing glaucoma.

Risk Factors for Glaucoma

Glaucoma is a complex eye condition that can lead to irreversible vision loss if not detected and managed early. Understanding the risk factors associated with glaucoma is crucial for effective prevention and early intervention.

Several demographic and genetic factors play a significant role in determining an individual's likelihood of developing this condition. Age is one of the most prominent risk factors; individuals over the age of 60 are at a higher risk, with the incidence increasing dramatically with advancing age.

Additionally, family history is a critical consideration; if a close relative has been diagnosed with glaucoma, the risk of developing the disease increases significantly, highlighting the importance of genetic predisposition.

Ethnicity also influences the likelihood of developing glaucoma, with certain groups being more susceptible. For example, people of African descent are at a higher risk for developing open-angle glaucoma, and they tend to experience more severe forms of the disease. In contrast, individuals of Asian descent may be more prone to angle-closure glaucoma.

Recognizing these ethnic variations in risk can help individuals take proactive steps in monitoring their eye health and seeking regular eye examinations, particularly if they belong to high-risk groups.

In addition to demographic factors, various medical conditions can elevate the risk of developing glaucoma. Conditions such as diabetes, high blood pressure, and heart disease have been linked to increased intraocular pressure, a key factor in the development of glaucoma.

Furthermore, those with a history of eye injuries or surgeries may also be at greater risk, as trauma can alter the normal functioning of the eye and its pressure regulation mechanisms. Individuals with these underlying health issues should be particularly vigilant about their eye care and maintain regular check-ups with their eye care professionals.

Certain lifestyle factors can also contribute to the risk of glaucoma. For instance, prolonged use of corticosteroid medications, whether systemic or topical, has been associated with increased intraocular pressure. Additionally, sedentary lifestyles that lack physical activity have been linked to higher rates of glaucoma.

Maintaining a healthy lifestyle through regular exercise, a balanced diet, and avoiding harmful substances such as tobacco can help mitigate these risks. Awareness of how lifestyle choices impact eye health is an essential component of a proactive prevention strategy.

Finally, understanding the importance of regular eye examinations cannot be overstated. Many individuals with glaucoma may not experience noticeable symptoms until significant damage has occurred. Routine eye exams that include measurements of intraocular pressure and thorough evaluations of the optic nerve can aid in early detection.

Individuals at higher risk should prioritize these exams and discuss their family history and any other risk factors with their eye care provider. Taking these proactive steps can significantly enhance the chances of preserving vision and maintaining overall eye health.

Symptoms and Early Detection

Symptoms of glaucoma can often be subtle and may not be immediately noticeable, which is why early detection is crucial. Most forms of glaucoma, particularly open-angle glaucoma, are asymptomatic in the early stages. Individuals may not experience any changes in their vision until significant damage has occurred. This lack of early symptoms can lead to the condition being undetected for years, highlighting the importance of regular eye examinations as a preventive measure.

In contrast, some types of glaucoma, such as acute angle-closure glaucoma, can present with more pronounced symptoms. These may include sudden eye pain, headache, nausea, vomiting, blurred vision, and seeing halos around lights.

If these symptoms occur, it is considered a medical emergency, and immediate attention is necessary to prevent permanent vision loss. Recognizing these acute signs is essential for timely intervention and treatment.

Routine eye exams play a vital role in the early detection of glaucoma. During these exams, eye care professionals measure intraocular pressure, assess the optic nerve's health, and conduct peripheral vision tests.

These evaluations can identify changes in eye pressure and optic nerve damage before any noticeable symptoms develop. Individuals at higher risk, such as those with a family history of glaucoma, African Americans over age 40, and individuals with certain medical conditions like diabetes, should prioritize regular screenings.

Monitoring changes in vision is another important aspect of early detection. Individuals should be aware of any gradual loss of peripheral vision or difficulty seeing in low light. Keeping a journal of any visual disturbances can help track changes over time, providing valuable information to eye care professionals during examinations. Awareness of these changes can prompt individuals to seek professional advice sooner rather than later.

Finally, education about glaucoma and its symptoms can empower individuals to take proactive steps in their eye health. Understanding risk factors and being vigilant about vision changes can facilitate earlier detection and treatment.

By fostering a culture of awareness and preventive care, individuals can significantly reduce the risk of developing advanced glaucoma and its associated complications. Regular communication with healthcare providers and adherence to recommended screening schedules can be instrumental in safeguarding eye health.

How To Prevent Glaucoma

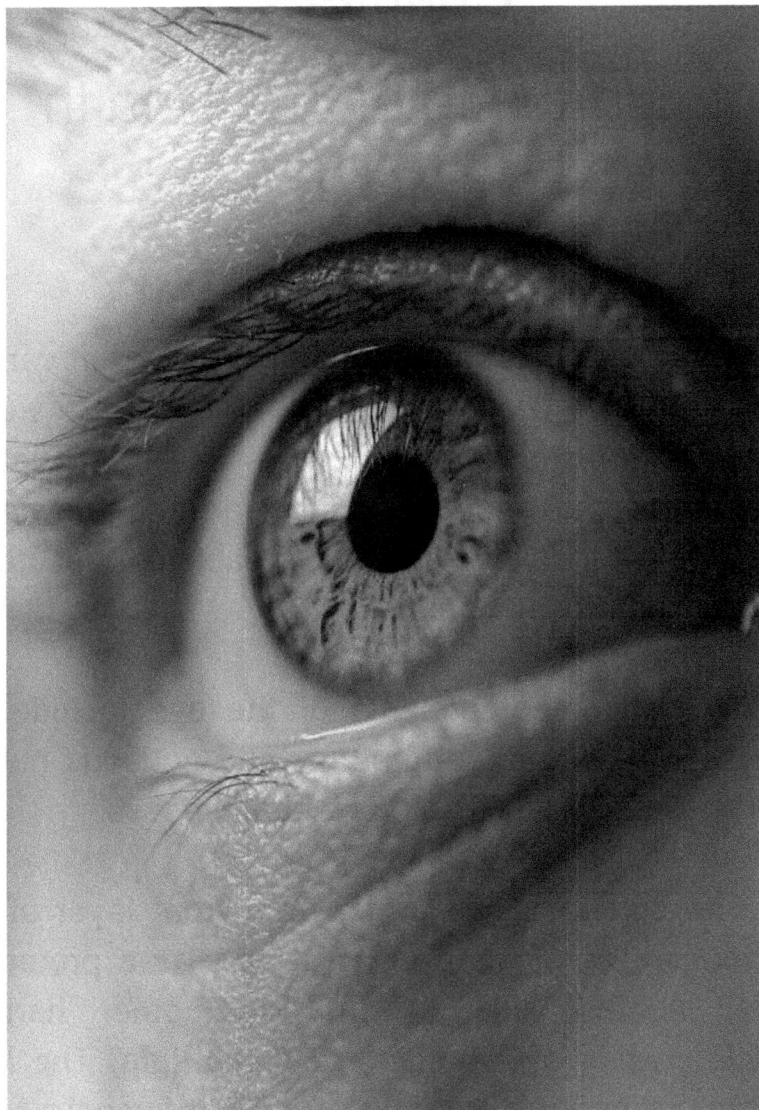

Chapter 2

Importance of Eye Health

The Anatomy of the Eye

The eye is a complex organ composed of various structures that work together to facilitate vision. Understanding the anatomy of the eye is crucial for those concerned about glaucoma, as this knowledge can empower individuals to take proactive measures in preserving their eye health.

The major components of the eye include the cornea, lens, retina, optic nerve, and aqueous humor, each playing a vital role in the visual process.

The cornea is the transparent front layer of the eye that allows light to enter. It acts as a protective barrier against dust, germs, and other harmful particles, while also helping to focus light. The lens, located just behind the cornea, further refines the focus of light onto the retina.

As people age, the lens can become less flexible, which may affect vision. For those at risk of glaucoma, maintaining the health of these structures is essential, as any changes can influence intraocular pressure and overall eye function.

The retina is a thin layer of tissue located at the back of the eye that converts light signals into electrical impulses. These impulses are transmitted to the brain via the optic nerve, allowing for the perception of images. In glaucoma, damage to the optic nerve can lead to vision loss, making it vital to understand how the retina and optic nerve interact. Regular eye exams can help detect changes in these areas, enabling early intervention and management of glaucoma.

Aqueous humor is a clear fluid produced by the eye that fills the space between the lens and the cornea. It plays a significant role in maintaining intraocular pressure, which is crucial for eye health. In glaucoma, the drainage of this fluid can be impaired, leading to increased pressure and potential damage to the optic nerve.

Understanding how aqueous humor production and drainage work is important for those looking to prevent glaucoma, as lifestyle choices and medical interventions can influence these processes.

In summary, a thorough comprehension of the eye's anatomy is essential for individuals concerned about glaucoma. By recognizing the functions and interconnections of the cornea, lens, retina, optic nerve, and aqueous humor, individuals can make informed decisions about their eye health. Furthermore, awareness of how changes in these structures can contribute to glaucoma underscores the importance of regular eye check-ups and proactive measures to maintain optimal eye function.

How Eye Pressure Affects Vision

Eye pressure, also known as intraocular pressure (IOP), plays a crucial role in maintaining the overall health of the eyes. It is determined by the balance between the production and drainage of the aqueous humor, the fluid found in the eye. When this balance is disrupted, it can lead to increased eye pressure, which is a significant risk factor for glaucoma.

Understanding how eye pressure affects vision is essential for those concerned about glaucoma and its potential impact on their sight.

Elevated eye pressure can lead to damage of the optic nerve, which is responsible for transmitting visual information from the eye to the brain. This damage often occurs gradually, making it difficult for individuals to recognize the problem until significant vision loss has occurred.

As the optic nerve deteriorates, the ability to see may diminish, often starting with peripheral vision. This gradual loss can go unnoticed until it reaches advanced stages, underscoring the importance of regular eye examinations for early detection.

The relationship between eye pressure and vision is complex, as not everyone with high eye pressure will develop glaucoma. Conversely, individuals with normal eye pressure can also experience optic nerve damage. This variability emphasizes the need for comprehensive eye assessments that go beyond simply measuring IOP.

Factors such as the health of the optic nerve, the thickness of the cornea, and individual risk factors must be evaluated to provide a complete picture of eye health.

Monitoring eye pressure is critical for preventing glaucoma and preserving vision. Regular check-ups with an eye care professional can help detect changes in IOP and identify any potential issues before they escalate. If elevated eye pressure is detected, various treatment options are available, including medications, laser treatments, and surgical interventions. These treatments aim to lower eye pressure and protect the optic nerve, thereby reducing the risk of vision loss.

In conclusion, understanding how eye pressure affects vision is vital for individuals concerned about glaucoma. By being proactive and engaging in regular eye care, it is possible to monitor eye health effectively and take necessary steps to prevent the onset of glaucoma. Awareness of the risks associated with elevated eye pressure can empower individuals to seek timely intervention, ultimately safeguarding their vision for the future.

The Role of the Optometrist and Ophthalmologist

The roles of optometrists and ophthalmologists are crucial in the prevention, diagnosis, and management of glaucoma. Optometrists are primary eye care providers who perform comprehensive eye examinations, assess visual acuity, and detect various eye conditions, including glaucoma.

They are trained to measure intraocular pressure, conduct visual field tests, and examine the optic nerve for early signs of glaucoma. By identifying risk factors and early symptoms, optometrists can recommend appropriate treatment options or refer patients to ophthalmologists for more specialized care.

Ophthalmologists, on the other hand, are medical doctors specializing in eye and vision care, including performing surgical procedures. They have a broader scope of practice compared to optometrists and can provide more advanced treatments for glaucoma, such as laser therapy or surgical interventions.

After an optometrist identifies a potential glaucoma case, they may refer the patient to an ophthalmologist for further evaluation and management. This collaborative approach ensures that patients receive comprehensive care tailored to their specific needs.

Both optometrists and ophthalmologists play a significant role in patient education regarding glaucoma. They inform patients about the importance of regular eye exams, particularly for those at increased risk, such as individuals with a family history of glaucoma, those over 40 years old, and people with certain medical conditions like diabetes.

Educating patients about the nature of glaucoma, its potential impact on vision, and the importance of adhering to prescribed treatments can empower individuals to take proactive steps in managing their eye health.

Regular follow-ups with either an optometrist or ophthalmologist are essential for monitoring eye health, especially for patients diagnosed with glaucoma. During these visits, eye care professionals can assess the effectiveness of treatment plans, adjust medications if necessary, and conduct ongoing tests to monitor the progression of the disease. This proactive management helps to preserve vision and prevent irreversible damage caused by glaucoma.

In conclusion, understanding the distinct yet complementary roles of optometrists and ophthalmologists is vital for anyone concerned about glaucoma.

By working together, these professionals provide comprehensive eye care that emphasizes early detection and effective management strategies. Individuals should prioritize regular eye examinations and take advantage of the expertise offered by both optometrists and ophthalmologists as part of their action plan for maintaining healthy eyes and preventing glaucoma.

How To Prevent Glaucoma

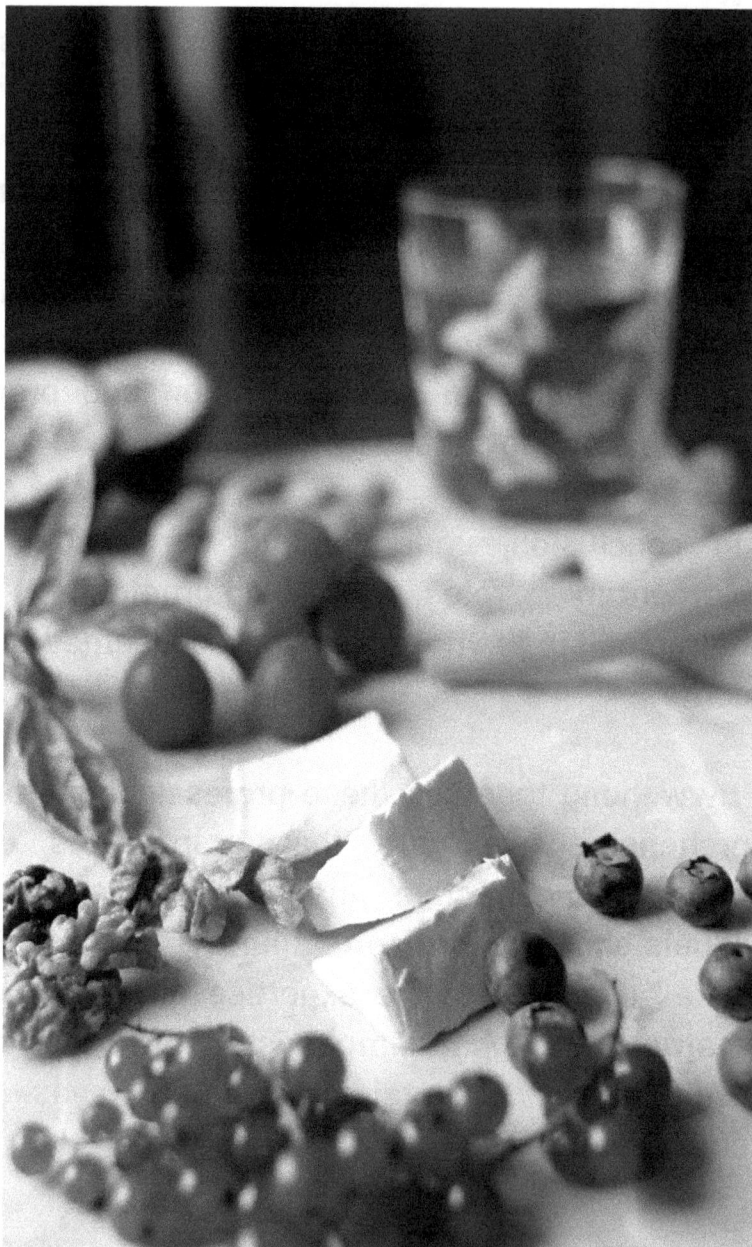

Chapter 3

Lifestyle Changes to Prevent Glaucoma

Diet and Nutrition

Diet and nutrition play a crucial role in maintaining overall eye health and may significantly influence the risk of developing glaucoma. A well-balanced diet rich in antioxidants, vitamins, and minerals can help protect the eyes from oxidative stress and inflammation, which are linked to various eye diseases, including glaucoma.

Consuming a variety of fruits and vegetables, particularly those high in vitamins A, C, and E, is essential. These nutrients are known for their ability to neutralize free radicals, thereby reducing the risk of eye damage.

Omega-3 fatty acids, commonly found in fish such as salmon, mackerel, and sardines, are another vital component of a diet aimed at preventing glaucoma. These fatty acids have anti-inflammatory properties and are believed to play a protective role in maintaining eye health. Incorporating sources of omega-3s into your meals can enhance retinal function and may help lower intraocular pressure, a significant risk factor for glaucoma.

For those who do not consume fish, walnuts, flaxseeds, and chia seeds serve as excellent plant-based alternatives.

Maintaining a healthy weight is also critical in preventing glaucoma. Obesity is associated with an increased risk of developing various health issues, including elevated intraocular pressure. A diet that promotes weight management should focus on whole grains, lean proteins, and healthy fats while limiting processed foods high in sugar and saturated fats. Regular physical activity, combined with a balanced diet, can help maintain a healthy weight and reduce the risk of glaucoma.

Hydration is often overlooked when discussing diet and eye health. Adequate water intake is essential for maintaining optimal eye function, as dehydration can lead to dry eyes and potentially exacerbate glaucoma symptoms. Aim to drink enough water throughout the day, and consider incorporating hydrating foods such as cucumbers, oranges, and lettuce into your diet. These foods not only contribute to hydration but also provide essential nutrients for overall health.

Finally, it is crucial to limit the intake of caffeine and alcohol, as excessive consumption of these substances can negatively affect intraocular pressure and overall eye health. Moderation is key; consuming these drinks in small amounts may not pose a significant risk.

However, being mindful of your intake and making healthier choices can contribute to better eye health. By focusing on a nutrient-rich diet and making informed dietary choices, individuals can take significant steps toward preventing glaucoma and promoting long-term eye wellness.

Exercise and Physical Activity

Exercise and physical activity play a crucial role in maintaining overall eye health, particularly in the prevention of glaucoma. Regular physical activity can help lower intraocular pressure (IOP), a key factor associated with glaucoma. Studies have shown that moderate exercise, such as walking, cycling, or swimming, can lead to a reduction in IOP, potentially decreasing the risk of developing glaucoma.

Engaging in these activities not only benefits the eyes but also contributes to better cardiovascular health, which is important since conditions like high blood pressure can further exacerbate eye problems.

Incorporating exercise into your daily routine does not require a complete overhaul of your lifestyle. Simple changes, such as taking the stairs instead of the elevator or setting aside time for a daily walk, can accumulate significant health benefits over time. It is recommended to aim for at least 150 minutes of moderate aerobic activity each week.

This can be broken down into manageable sessions, making it easier to fit into a busy schedule. Consistency is key; establishing a routine will help ensure that physical activity becomes a lasting part of your life.

Strength training is another important aspect of a well-rounded exercise regimen. While aerobic exercises are vital for maintaining heart health and lowering IOP, resistance training can enhance overall muscle strength and endurance.

This type of exercise can also improve balance and coordination, reducing the risk of falls and injuries, which is particularly important as one ages. Incorporating strength training exercises two to three times per week can complement aerobic activities and contribute to overall physical health.

Engaging in mind-body exercises, such as yoga and tai chi, can also be beneficial for those concerned about glaucoma. These practices not only promote relaxation and stress reduction but also improve flexibility and balance. Some studies suggest that certain yoga poses can help decrease IOP.

Additionally, the meditative aspects of these exercises can contribute to overall mental well-being, which is essential in managing chronic conditions like glaucoma. Mind-body exercises can be a gentle yet effective way to stay active while also addressing stress, which may impact eye health.

Before starting any new exercise program, it is advisable to consult with a healthcare professional, especially for individuals with pre-existing health conditions or those who have not been active for some time. They can provide personalized recommendations and ensure that the chosen activities are safe and appropriate.

By prioritizing regular exercise and physical activity, individuals concerned about glaucoma can take significant steps toward preserving their eye health and enhancing their quality of life.

Maintaining a Healthy Weight

Maintaining a healthy weight is crucial not only for overall well-being but also for the prevention of glaucoma. Research has indicated that obesity can increase the risk of developing glaucoma, particularly primary open-angle glaucoma. Excess weight can lead to elevated intraocular pressure (IOP), which is a significant risk factor for this eye condition. Therefore, understanding the link between weight management and eye health is essential for individuals concerned about glaucoma.

To effectively maintain a healthy weight, it is important to adopt a balanced diet rich in fruits, vegetables, whole grains, and lean proteins. Foods that are high in antioxidants, such as leafy greens and berries, can contribute to eye health by reducing oxidative stress.

Additionally, incorporating omega-3 fatty acids found in fish can support overall ocular health. Avoiding processed foods, excessive sugar, and high-fat snacks can help manage weight and, in turn, may reduce the risk of elevated IOP.

Physical activity plays a vital role in weight management and is equally important in preventing glaucoma. Regular exercise helps to burn calories, reduces stress, and improves circulation, which can positively affect eye pressure.

Engaging in activities such as walking, swimming, or cycling for at least 150 minutes per week can help maintain a healthy weight. Individuals should choose activities they enjoy to ensure consistency and make exercise a regular part of their lifestyle.

In addition to diet and exercise, monitoring weight regularly can help individuals stay on track with their health goals. Keeping a journal of food intake and physical activity can provide insights into patterns and areas for improvement.

Setting realistic and achievable weight loss or maintenance goals can motivate individuals to stay committed. Moreover, seeking support from healthcare providers or nutritionists can provide personalized guidance tailored to specific needs and concerns related to glaucoma.

Finally, maintaining a healthy weight is a lifelong commitment that requires ongoing effort and awareness. Regular eye examinations are crucial for those at risk of glaucoma, as early detection can lead to better management of the condition. By prioritizing weight management, individuals can not only enhance their overall health but also take proactive steps in reducing their risk of glaucoma, ensuring better eye health for years to come.

How To Prevent Glaucoma

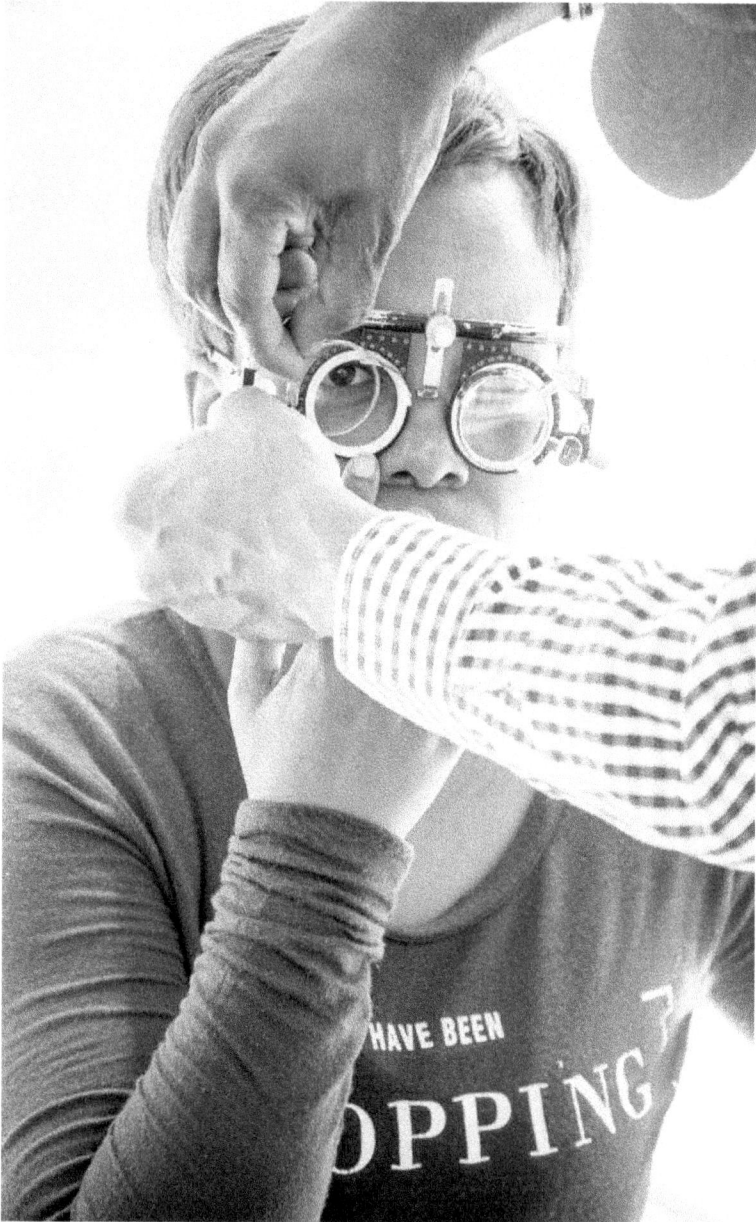

Chapter 4

Regular Eye Exams

The Importance of Routine Eye Check-ups

Routine eye check-ups play a crucial role in the early detection and prevention of glaucoma, a condition that can lead to irreversible vision loss if not addressed promptly. Regular visits to an eye care professional allow for comprehensive examinations that can identify changes in eye pressure, optic nerve health, and visual field function.

These assessments are essential because glaucoma often develops without noticeable symptoms until significant damage has occurred. By prioritizing routine eye check-ups, individuals can catch potential issues early and take proactive steps to protect their vision.

During an eye examination, an ophthalmologist or optometrist can utilize various diagnostic tools to measure intraocular pressure, which is a key factor in glaucoma risk. Tonometry is one such method, helping to determine if the pressure in the eye is within a healthy range.

Elevated intraocular pressure is one of the primary indicators of glaucoma, although not everyone with high pressure will develop the disease. Regular monitoring allows for the timely detection of pressure fluctuations and enables healthcare providers to tailor preventive strategies based on individual risk profiles.

In addition to measuring eye pressure, routine check-ups include assessments of the optic nerve and peripheral vision. These evaluations can reveal early signs of glaucoma damage, which is crucial, as the condition can progress silently. The optic nerve head is examined using techniques such as optic coherence tomography (OCT) or fundus photography.

These advanced imaging technologies provide detailed views of the nerve fibers and can help identify subtle changes that may indicate the onset of glaucoma. Early intervention can be vital in managing the disease and preserving vision.

For individuals at higher risk of developing glaucoma, such as those with a family history of the disease, diabetes, or hypertension, routine eye check-ups become even more essential. These individuals should consult their eye care provider about how often they should be screened.

The American Academy of Ophthalmology recommends that adults aged 40 and older have a comprehensive eye exam every one to two years, with more frequent evaluations for those at increased risk. Establishing a routine schedule can help ensure that any potential issues are addressed promptly.

Finally, patient education during eye check-ups is invaluable for empowering individuals to take charge of their eye health. Eye care professionals can provide guidance on lifestyle choices that may reduce the risk of glaucoma, such as maintaining a healthy diet, exercising regularly, and avoiding smoking.

Moreover, they can discuss the importance of adhering to prescribed treatments if glaucoma is diagnosed. By fostering an ongoing dialogue about eye health, routine check-ups can play a pivotal role in preventing glaucoma and ensuring that individuals maintain their vision for years to come.

What to Expect During an Eye Exam

An eye exam is a crucial step in maintaining eye health and preventing conditions like glaucoma. During this examination, the eye care professional will assess various aspects of your vision and eye health. You can expect a series of tests designed to evaluate your vision clarity, eye pressure, and overall eye function. Being informed about what to expect can help alleviate any anxiety and ensure that you are prepared for your appointment.

The examination typically begins with a review of your medical history and any symptoms you may be experiencing. It's essential to discuss any family history of eye diseases, especially glaucoma, as this can influence your risk level.

Your eye care provider will ask about medications you are taking and any previous eye treatments. This information helps them tailor the exam to your specific needs and risk factors.

Following the history review, your eye care provider will conduct a visual acuity test. This test measures how well you can see at various distances, usually using an eye chart. You will be asked to read letters from a distance to determine the clarity of your vision. Additionally, a refraction test might be performed to determine if you need corrective lenses. This initial assessment is vital, as visual acuity can be an early indicator of potential problems, including glaucoma.

Next, the doctor will measure your intraocular pressure (IOP), which is a key factor in glaucoma detection. This test is typically performed using a tonometer, which gently flattens the surface of your eye to measure the pressure inside. Elevated IOP can be a warning sign for glaucoma, making this test especially important for individuals concerned about the disease. Depending on the findings, further tests may be recommended to assess the health of your optic nerve and the drainage angle of your eye.

Finally, your eye care provider may conduct additional tests such as a visual field test or optical coherence tomography (OCT) to evaluate the peripheral vision and the health of the optic nerve. These tests provide valuable information about the functioning of your eyes and can help detect any early signs of glaucoma.

Understanding what to expect during an eye exam can empower you to take an active role in your eye health, making it easier to detect and prevent glaucoma before it leads to significant vision loss.

Frequency of Eye Exams Based on Risk

Regular eye examinations are essential for everyone, but they become increasingly important for individuals at higher risk for glaucoma. The frequency of these exams can vary based on several factors, including age, family history, and the presence of other medical conditions. For those concerned about glaucoma, understanding when and how often to get their eyes checked can play a crucial role in prevention and early detection.

For individuals with no known risk factors, such as a family history of glaucoma, the general recommendation is to have a comprehensive eye exam every two years. However, as people reach the age of 40, they should consider increasing the frequency of their visits to once a year.

This change is vital because the likelihood of developing glaucoma increases with age, and early detection can significantly improve treatment outcomes.

Those with a family history of glaucoma are advised to have their eyes examined more frequently. If a close relative has been diagnosed with glaucoma, it is recommended to begin regular eye exams at the age of 30. In this case, annual exams are suggested to monitor eye pressure and assess the optic nerve for any signs of damage.

This proactive approach is crucial, as genetic predisposition can significantly elevate the risk of developing the disease.

Individuals with other medical conditions, such as diabetes or hypertension, are also at an increased risk for glaucoma. For these patients, comprehensive eye exams should occur at least once a year, regardless of their age. Diabetes can lead to changes in the eye that may contribute to glaucoma, while high blood pressure can affect blood flow to the optic nerve. Regular monitoring by an eye care professional can help mitigate these risks.

In summary, the frequency of eye exams based on risk factors should be tailored to each individual's circumstances. Those with no risk factors should have eye exams every two years until age 40, after which annual exams are advisable. Individuals with a family history of glaucoma or other medical conditions should prioritize yearly examinations.

By adhering to these recommendations, individuals can take proactive steps in preventing glaucoma and ensuring long-term eye health.

How To Prevent Glaucoma

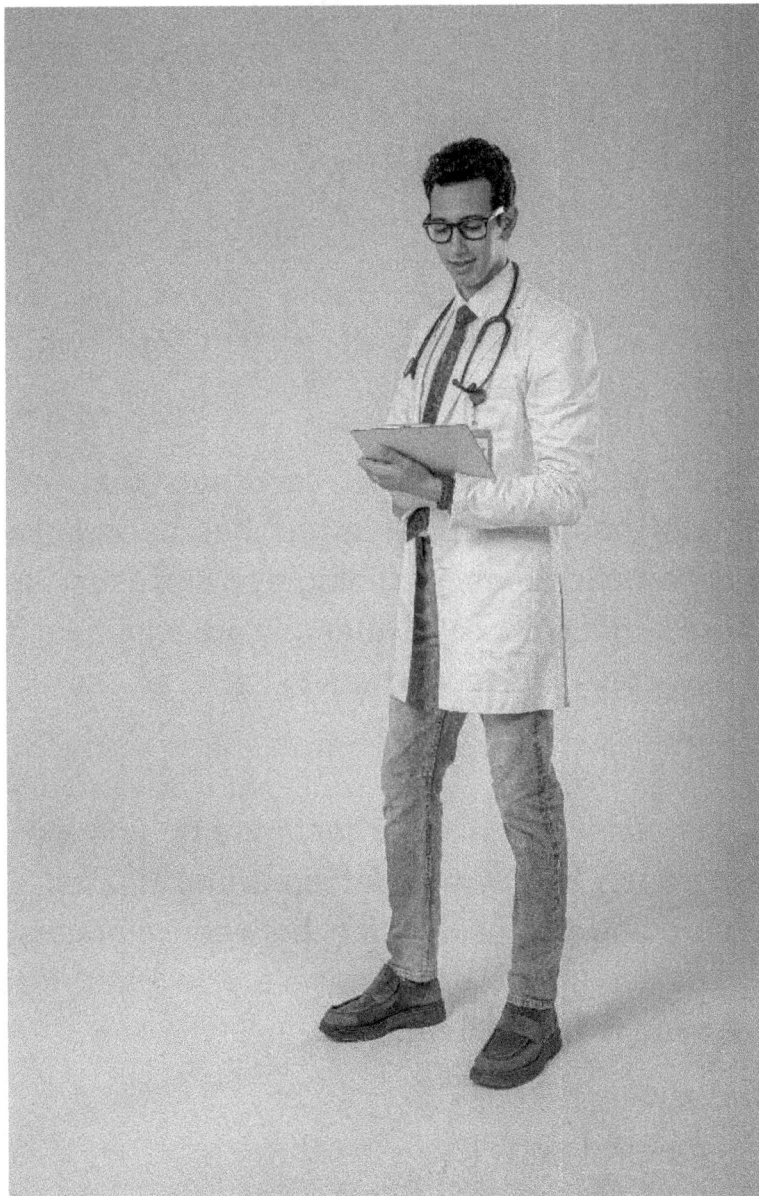

Your Action Plan for Healthy Eyes

Chapter 5

Managing Health Conditions

The Connection Between Diabetes and Glaucoma

Diabetes is a chronic condition that affects millions of people worldwide and has been linked to various complications, including eye diseases. One of the more serious concerns that can arise in individuals with diabetes is the increased risk of developing glaucoma.

This condition, which affects the optic nerve, can lead to vision loss if not detected and treated early. Understanding the connection between diabetes and glaucoma is crucial for those who are concerned about maintaining their eye health.

Research indicates that individuals with diabetes are at a higher risk of developing open-angle glaucoma, the most common form of the disease. The mechanisms behind this connection are multifaceted. Elevated blood sugar levels can contribute to changes in the eye's drainage system, leading to increased intraocular pressure (IOP).

This increased pressure can damage the optic nerve over time, which is a significant risk factor for glaucoma. Additionally, diabetic retinopathy, a common complication of diabetes, can also influence the development of glaucoma, further complicating the eye health of diabetic patients.

Managing diabetes effectively is essential in reducing the risk of glaucoma. Keeping blood sugar levels stable through a balanced diet, regular exercise, and adherence to prescribed medications can help mitigate the potential complications associated with diabetes. Regular eye examinations are also vital for those with diabetes. Eye care professionals can monitor changes in the eyes and catch early signs of glaucoma, enabling timely interventions that can preserve vision.

Symptoms of glaucoma often develop gradually, making routine screenings even more critical for people with diabetes. Many individuals may not experience noticeable symptoms until significant damage has occurred.

Therefore, it is recommended that people with diabetes have comprehensive eye exams at least once a year, or more frequently if advised by an eye care specialist. Early detection and treatment of glaucoma can significantly improve outcomes and help maintain eye health.

In conclusion, the link between diabetes and glaucoma underscores the importance of proactive health management. By understanding the risks and maintaining regular check-ups, individuals can take significant steps toward preventing glaucoma and safeguarding their vision.

Education on both diabetes management and the importance of eye health is essential for those who are concerned about glaucoma, ensuring they are well-equipped to make informed decisions regarding their care.

High Blood Pressure and Eye Health

High blood pressure, or hypertension, is a condition that can significantly impact overall health, including eye health. With the increasing prevalence of hypertension in modern society, understanding its implications for eye conditions, particularly glaucoma, is essential for individuals concerned about their vision.

High blood pressure can lead to changes in the blood vessels of the eyes, which may contribute to the development or exacerbation of glaucoma. This connection emphasizes the importance of monitoring blood pressure levels and managing them effectively to protect eye health.

The relationship between hypertension and glaucoma is complex. Elevated blood pressure can affect the optic nerve, which is critical for vision. When the optic nerve is damaged, it can lead to vision loss and, in severe cases, permanent blindness.

Moreover, high blood pressure can reduce the flow of blood to the optic nerve, depriving it of the oxygen and nutrients necessary for its proper functioning. This reduced blood flow can increase the risk of developing open-angle glaucoma, the most common form of the disease.

Regular eye examinations are vital for individuals with high blood pressure. During these check-ups, eye care professionals can assess the health of the optic nerve and look for signs of glaucoma. Early detection is crucial, as glaucoma often progresses without noticeable symptoms until significant damage has occurred.

Individuals with hypertension should discuss their blood pressure management strategies with their primary healthcare provider and ensure that their eye care provider is aware of their condition. This collaborative approach can help in early identification and intervention, reducing the risk of vision loss.

Lifestyle modifications play an essential role in managing high blood pressure and, by extension, protecting eye health. A balanced diet rich in fruits, vegetables, whole grains, and low-fat dairy can help maintain healthy blood pressure levels. Regular physical activity, weight management, and stress reduction techniques, such as mindfulness or yoga, can also contribute to better blood pressure control.

Additionally, limiting salt intake and avoiding tobacco use are important strategies for individuals concerned about both hypertension and glaucoma.

In conclusion, maintaining healthy blood pressure levels is crucial for preserving eye health, particularly for those at risk of glaucoma. Individuals should be proactive in monitoring their blood pressure and engaging in lifestyle changes that support cardiovascular health.

Regular eye examinations and open communication with healthcare providers can facilitate early detection of any potential issues, ensuring that appropriate measures are taken to safeguard vision.

By prioritizing both blood pressure management and eye health, individuals can take significant steps toward preventing glaucoma and maintaining their overall quality of life.

Other Conditions Impacting Eye Health

Several conditions can significantly impact eye health and potentially increase the risk of glaucoma. Understanding these conditions is crucial for individuals concerned about preserving their vision. Among the most notable are diabetes, hypertension, and ocular hypertension. Each of these conditions can alter intraocular pressure or damage the optic nerve, making it essential to monitor and manage them effectively.

Diabetes, particularly diabetic retinopathy, poses a significant threat to eye health. This condition arises when high blood sugar levels damage the blood vessels in the retina, leading to vision complications. Individuals with diabetes are at a higher risk of developing glaucoma due to changes in blood flow and pressure within the eye.

Regular eye examinations are critical for those with diabetes, allowing for early detection and timely management of any potential complications that may arise.

Hypertension, or high blood pressure, can also play a role in eye health. It can lead to damage of the blood vessels in the eyes, contributing to the development of glaucoma. Elevated blood pressure may increase the risk of optic nerve damage, making it vital for individuals with hypertension to regularly monitor their blood pressure and maintain it within healthy ranges.

Lifestyle changes such as diet and exercise, along with prescribed medications, can help manage hypertension and subsequently protect eye health.

Ocular hypertension is a condition characterized by elevated intraocular pressure without any detectable damage to the optic nerve or vision. While not everyone with ocular hypertension will develop glaucoma, this condition serves as a significant risk factor.

It is essential for individuals with ocular hypertension to undergo regular eye examinations to monitor pressure levels and optic nerve health. Early intervention can help prevent the onset of glaucoma, making awareness and proactive management key components of eye care.

In addition to these conditions, lifestyle factors such as smoking, obesity, and excessive alcohol consumption can further impact eye health. These habits can contribute to systemic health issues that may exacerbate the risk of glaucoma.

Adopting a healthy lifestyle through a balanced diet, regular physical activity, and avoiding harmful substances can significantly reduce the likelihood of developing conditions that threaten eye health. By being informed about these factors, individuals can take proactive steps to protect their vision and lower the risk of glaucoma.

How To Prevent Glaucoma

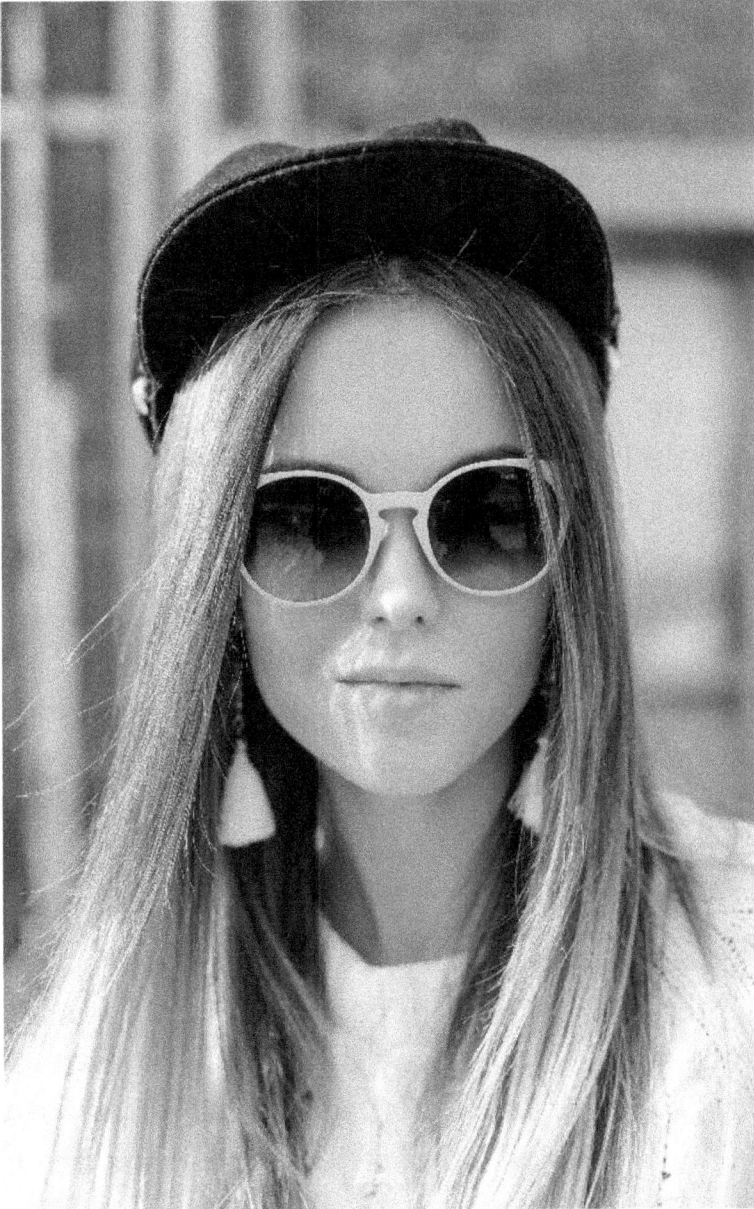

Chapter 6

Protecting Your Eyes

UV Protection and Sunglasses

Ultraviolet (UV) radiation from the sun can have detrimental effects on eye health, particularly for individuals concerned about glaucoma. Prolonged exposure to UV rays can contribute to the development of cataracts and other eye conditions that may exacerbate the risk of glaucoma.

Therefore, it is essential to understand the importance of UV protection and the role that sunglasses play in safeguarding your eyes from harmful radiation.

When selecting sunglasses, it is crucial to ensure they offer 100% UV protection. Not all sunglasses are created equal, and many may lack adequate UV filtering. Look for labels that specify UV400 or 100% UV protection, as these indicate that the lenses can block both UVA and UVB rays.

Additionally, polarized lenses can reduce glare, enhancing visual comfort and clarity, which is particularly beneficial for individuals with existing eye conditions.

Sunglasses should not only be a fashion accessory but also a critical component of your eye care routine. Wearing sunglasses can significantly reduce the amount of UV radiation that penetrates the eyes, thus lowering the risk of developing conditions that may lead to glaucoma. It is advisable to wear sunglasses whenever you are outdoors, even on cloudy days, as UV rays can penetrate through clouds and still pose a threat to your eye health.

In addition to sunglasses, wide-brimmed hats can provide extra protection by blocking sunlight from reaching your eyes. This combination of sunglasses and hats can create a barrier against harmful UV exposure, especially during peak sunlight hours when UV radiation is strongest.

By taking these precautions, you can enhance your overall eye protection and contribute to maintaining healthy vision.

Regular eye examinations are also vital for monitoring eye health and detecting any early signs of glaucoma. During these visits, your eye care professional can assess your risk factors and recommend appropriate measures, including UV protection strategies. Incorporating proper sunglasses into your daily routine, along with regular check-ups, can play a significant role in your proactive approach to preventing glaucoma and preserving your vision for the future.

Safety Measures in the Workplace

Safety measures in the workplace play a crucial role in preventing not only physical injuries but also health issues that could potentially lead to conditions like glaucoma. Individuals who are concerned about their eye health must recognize that their work environment can significantly influence their overall well-being.

Proper lighting, ergonomic workstations, and the use of protective eyewear are essential components of a safe workplace that can help mitigate the risk factors associated with glaucoma.

Adequate lighting is vital for reducing eye strain and preventing vision problems. Work areas should be well-lit, utilizing natural light whenever possible, as it is less harsh than fluorescent lighting.

Employees should also ensure that their workspaces are free from glare by positioning screens away from direct light sources. Incorporating adjustable lighting options allows individuals to customize their environment according to their needs, further promoting eye health and reducing the likelihood of developing conditions like glaucoma.

Ergonomics is another critical aspect of workplace safety that can impact eye health. A well-designed workstation can help reduce physical strain on the body, including the eyes.

This includes ensuring that computer screens are positioned at eye level and that chairs provide proper support. Taking regular breaks to rest the eyes and practicing the 20-20-20 rule—looking at something 20 feet away for 20 seconds every 20 minutes—can help alleviate eye fatigue.

By adopting ergonomic practices, employees can maintain better visual function and potentially lower their risk of developing glaucoma.

The use of protective eyewear is essential in environments where exposure to harmful substances or physical hazards is a concern. Safety goggles or glasses can protect the eyes from dust, chemicals, and flying debris, which can lead to injuries and long-term damage. For those working in industries such as construction or manufacturing, it is particularly important to use appropriate eye protection.

This not only safeguards against immediate eye injuries but also helps in preserving long-term eye health, which is vital for preventing glaucoma.

Lastly, fostering a culture of awareness and education about eye health among employees can further enhance workplace safety. Regular training sessions on the importance of eye care, the risks associated with glaucoma, and the implementation of safety measures can empower individuals to take proactive steps in protecting their vision.

Encouraging open communication about eye health concerns and providing resources for regular eye examinations can significantly contribute to early detection and prevention of glaucoma, ensuring that employees remain informed and vigilant about their eye health.

Avoiding Eye Injuries

Eye injuries can significantly impact overall eye health and may contribute to conditions like glaucoma. To prevent such injuries, it is essential to understand the different types of risks present in daily life. Common situations that can lead to eye injuries include exposure to hazardous substances, improper use of tools or machinery, and even recreational activities. Being aware of these risks is the first step towards safeguarding your eyes and maintaining optimal health.

Protective eyewear is one of the most effective ways to prevent eye injuries. Whether you are working in a factory, participating in sports, or engaging in home improvement projects, wearing safety goggles or glasses can shield your eyes from flying debris, chemicals, and other potential hazards.

It is crucial to select the appropriate type of eyewear for specific activities; for example, impact-resistant lenses are important for construction work, while UV-blocking sunglasses are necessary for outdoor activities. Investing in high-quality protective eyewear can significantly reduce the risk of injury.

In addition to wearing protective gear, maintaining a safe environment is vital for preventing eye injuries. This includes organizing workspaces to minimize clutter, using tools properly, and ensuring that hazardous materials are stored safely. In homes with children, it is essential to teach them about the dangers of sharp objects and the importance of being cautious around chemicals. Regularly inspecting your surroundings for potential hazards can help create a safer environment for everyone.

Education and awareness play a critical role in preventing eye injuries. Understanding the symptoms of eye injuries, such as pain, redness, or vision changes, can prompt immediate action if an incident occurs. It is essential to know first aid steps, such as flushing the eye with clean water in case of chemical exposure or covering the eye with a clean cloth if there is an injury.

Promptly seeking professional medical attention can prevent long-term damage and complications, including those that may worsen the risk of glaucoma.

Lastly, regular eye examinations are crucial for early detection of any potential issues that could lead to glaucoma and other eye conditions. During these visits, eye care professionals can assess your eye health, provide guidance on injury prevention, and recommend protective measures tailored to your lifestyle. Staying proactive about your eye health not only helps you avoid injuries but also ensures that you maintain the best possible vision and reduce the risk of developing glaucoma in the future.

How To Prevent Glaucoma

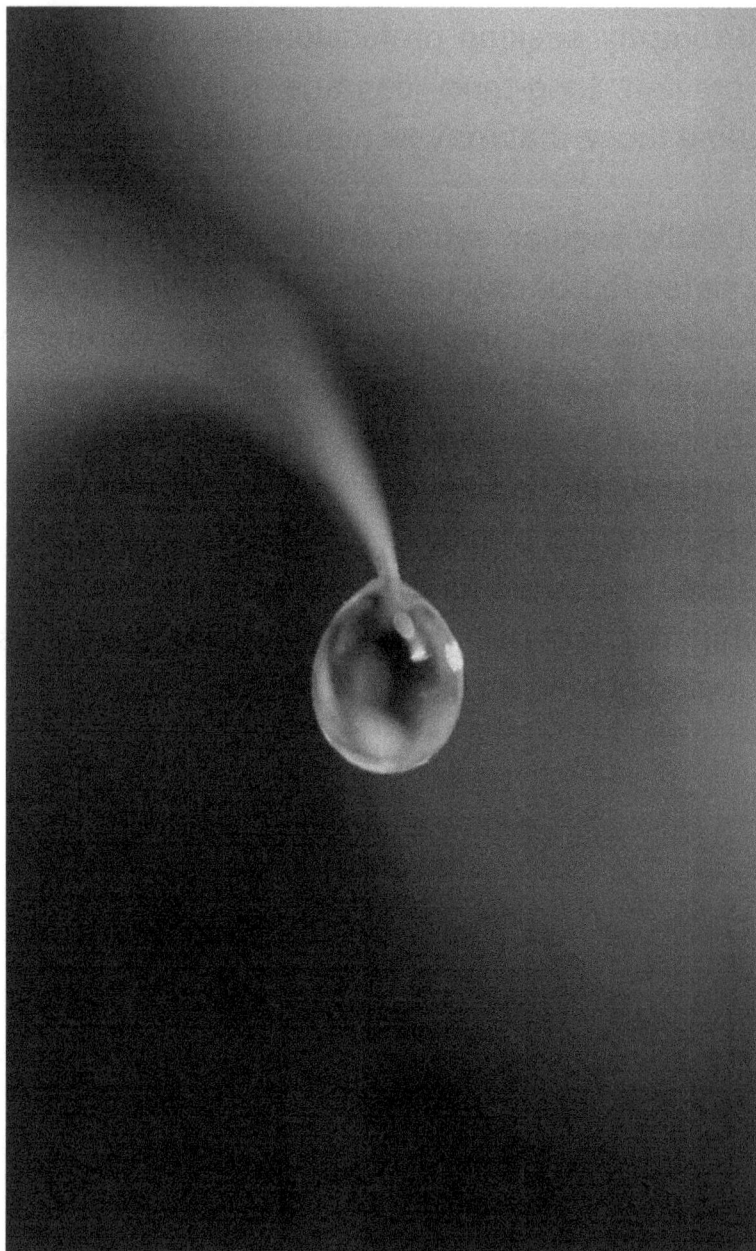

Your Action Plan for Healthy Eyes

Chapter 7

Medications and Treatments

Eye Drops and Their Role in Prevention

Eye drops play a crucial role in the prevention and management of glaucoma, a condition that can lead to irreversible vision loss if left untreated. These medications are designed to lower intraocular pressure (IOP), which is a significant risk factor for glaucoma.

By reducing IOP, eye drops can help protect the optic nerve from damage, thus preserving vision. For individuals concerned about glaucoma, understanding the types of eye drops available and their proper use is essential for maintaining eye health.

There are several classes of eye drops used in the treatment of glaucoma, each working through different mechanisms to lower IOP.

Prostaglandin analogs are among the most commonly prescribed; they increase the outflow of fluid from the eye, thereby reducing pressure. Beta-blockers are another class that decreases the production of fluid within the eye. Alpha agonists, carbonic anhydrase inhibitors, and Rho kinase inhibitors also contribute to IOP reduction through various pathways.

Knowing these options allows patients to engage in informed discussions with their eye care professionals about the most suitable treatment for their specific condition.

Consistency in using prescribed eye drops is vital for their effectiveness. Patients should adhere to the prescribed schedule, as regular use can significantly impact the management of IOP. Missing doses can lead to fluctuations in pressure, increasing the risk of optic nerve damage.

For those who struggle with remembering to take their medication, strategies such as setting reminders on smartphones or integrating the drops into daily routines can help.

Additionally, understanding the correct technique for applying eye drops can enhance their efficacy, ensuring that the medication reaches the intended site of action.

Regular follow-ups with an eye care professional are crucial for individuals using glaucoma eye drops. These appointments allow for monitoring of IOP levels and assessment of the treatment's effectiveness. Adjustments may be necessary if IOP remains high or if the patient experiences side effects from the medication.

Open communication between patients and healthcare providers fosters a collaborative approach to managing glaucoma, ensuring that any concerns are addressed promptly and that treatment plans remain aligned with the patient's needs.

Beyond their immediate role in lowering IOP, eye drops also serve as a preventive measure against the progression of glaucoma. For individuals at higher risk, such as those with a family history of the disease or other underlying health conditions, proactive management through eye drops can be a key strategy in reducing the likelihood of vision loss.

By understanding the importance of these medications and committing to their use, patients can take significant steps toward protecting their vision and maintaining their quality of life.

Understanding Surgical Options

Surgical intervention for glaucoma is often considered when other treatment methods, such as medications and laser therapies, fail to adequately control intraocular pressure (IOP). The primary goal of any surgical procedure in glaucoma management is to lower IOP and preserve the visual field.

It is essential for those at risk of glaucoma to understand the various surgical options available, as well as the potential benefits and risks associated with each procedure. This knowledge can empower patients to make informed decisions about their treatment plans.

One common surgical option is trabeculectomy, which involves creating a new drainage pathway for aqueous humor, the fluid inside the eye.

During this procedure, a small piece of tissue is removed from the sclera, allowing the fluid to bypass the blocked drainage system and flow directly into a space created under the conjunctiva. This can significantly lower IOP, but it does come with potential complications such as infection or scarring, which may affect the success of the surgery. Patients should engage in thorough discussions with their ophthalmologists to weigh the likelihood of success against these risks.

Another innovative approach is the use of minimally invasive glaucoma surgeries (MIGS). These procedures are designed to lower IOP with reduced trauma to the eye, leading to quicker recovery times and fewer complications. MIGS techniques include the placement of small devices that enhance fluid drainage or the use of microincisions to facilitate aqueous humor outflow.

While MIGS is generally safer than traditional surgical methods, they may not be suitable for all types of glaucoma. Understanding the specifics of each MIGS option can help patients determine if they are viable candidates.

For those with advanced glaucoma, more extensive surgical techniques such as tube shunt surgery may be considered. This procedure involves implanting a small tube that drains fluid from the eye into a reservoir, effectively managing IOP. Tube shunt surgery is particularly useful for patients who have not responded well to other treatments.

However, it also carries risks, including the potential for tube-related complications and the need for long-term follow-up care. A discussion with a glaucoma specialist can help patients assess whether tube shunt surgery aligns with their individual needs.

Ultimately, the choice of surgical intervention should be tailored to the specific type and severity of glaucoma, as well as the patient's overall health and lifestyle. Regular consultations with an eye care professional can provide ongoing assessments and recommendations as treatment options evolve. Understanding the surgical landscape of glaucoma management allows patients to engage actively in their care and take steps toward maintaining their eye health, potentially reducing the risk of vision loss associated with this condition.

Alternative Therapies

Alternative therapies offer various approaches to managing eye health and may serve as complementary options for individuals concerned about glaucoma. While traditional medical treatments are essential in managing this condition, many people seek additional methods to support their overall eye health. Understanding these therapies can empower patients to make informed choices and enhance their well-being.

One popular alternative therapy is acupuncture, an ancient practice rooted in Traditional Chinese Medicine. Proponents of acupuncture believe that it may help improve circulation and reduce intraocular pressure, which is crucial for glaucoma management.

Although scientific evidence on its effectiveness is still limited, some studies suggest that acupuncture may provide relief from symptoms associated with eye strain and fatigue. Before pursuing acupuncture, individuals should consult with their healthcare provider to ensure it aligns with their overall treatment plan.

Another alternative therapy gaining attention is the use of nutritional supplements. Certain vitamins and minerals, such as omega-3 fatty acids, vitamin A, and antioxidants, are thought to support eye health. Research indicates that a diet rich in these nutrients might help reduce the risk of developing glaucoma and other eye conditions.

Incorporating foods such as leafy greens, fatty fish, nuts, and berries into one's diet can be beneficial. However, it is crucial to discuss any supplement regimen with a healthcare professional to avoid potential interactions with prescribed medications.

Mind-body practices, including yoga and meditation, are also considered alternative therapies for maintaining eye health. These practices promote relaxation and reduce stress, which may indirectly benefit individuals with glaucoma. Stress has been linked to increased intraocular pressure, so adopting mindfulness techniques can serve as a preventive measure.

Additionally, specific yoga poses are believed to improve blood circulation to the eyes, contributing to better overall eye health. Engaging in these practices regularly can foster a holistic approach to managing glaucoma.

Herbal remedies are another avenue some individuals explore for eye health. Herbs such as bilberry and ginkgo biloba are often touted for their potential benefits in improving vision and circulation. However, scientific support for their effectiveness in preventing or treating glaucoma is still emerging.

As with any alternative therapy, individuals should exercise caution and consult with a healthcare provider before incorporating herbal supplements into their regimen. This ensures safety and compatibility with existing treatments, allowing for a well-rounded approach to eye health.

How To Prevent Glaucoma

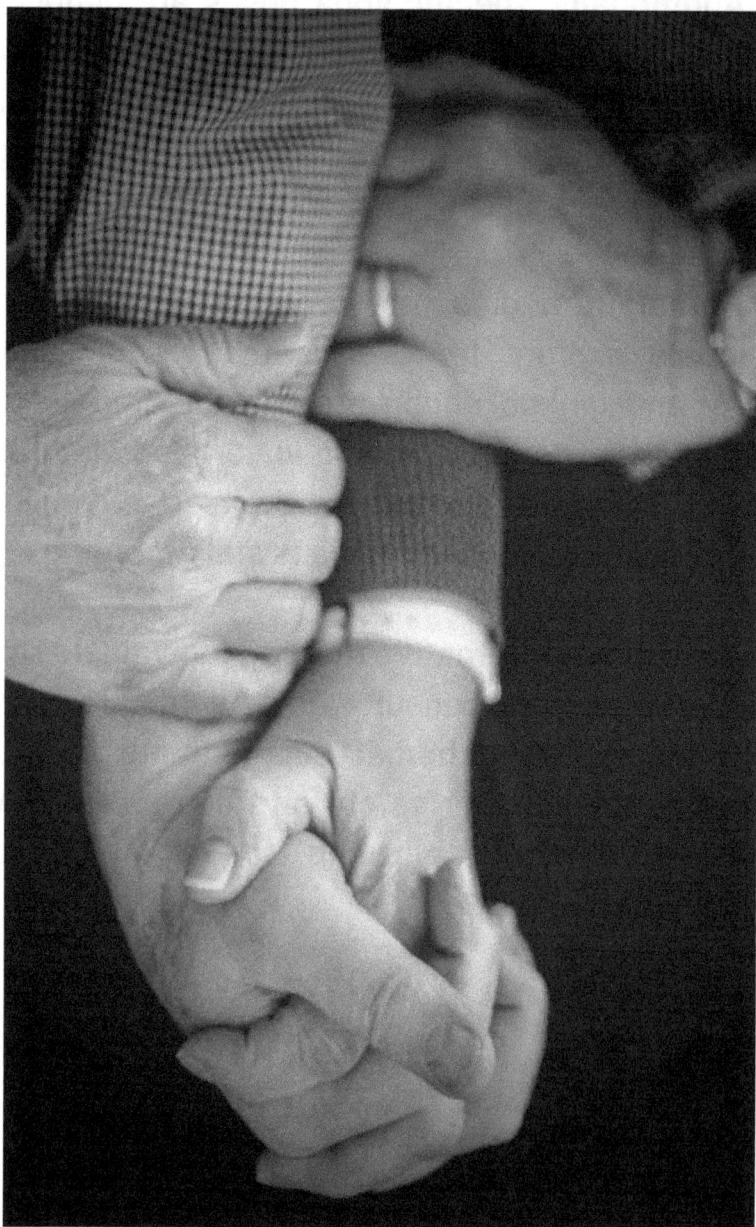

Chapter 8

Staying Informed

Resources for Glaucoma Awareness

Glaucoma awareness is crucial for early detection and effective management of the disease. Numerous resources are available to individuals seeking information about glaucoma, its risk factors, preventive measures, and treatment options.

Organizations such as the American Academy of Ophthalmology and the Glaucoma Research Foundation provide comprehensive educational materials, including brochures, videos, and online resources.

These organizations also offer access to recent research findings and clinical trials, helping individuals stay informed about advancements in glaucoma care.

Local health departments and community health organizations often host workshops and seminars focused on eye health and glaucoma prevention. Attending these events can provide valuable opportunities to learn from healthcare professionals, ask questions, and connect with others who share similar concerns.

Many eye care professionals also engage in outreach efforts by providing free screenings and informational sessions, ensuring that individuals have access to essential eye health resources in their communities.

Online platforms play a significant role in spreading glaucoma awareness. Websites dedicated to eye health, such as the National Eye Institute, offer a wealth of information on glaucoma symptoms, risk factors, and lifestyle changes that can contribute to eye health. Social media campaigns and online support groups can connect individuals facing glaucoma challenges, fostering a sense of community and shared experiences.

Engaging with these platforms can help people stay motivated and informed about their eye health.

Educational materials specifically designed for various demographics are also available. For instance, resources tailored for seniors often address age-related concerns and emphasize the importance of regular eye exams.

Additionally, materials aimed at caregivers can enhance their understanding of glaucoma, allowing them to support their loved ones effectively. Ensuring that these resources are accessible and relevant to different audiences is vital in promoting awareness and encouraging proactive health measures.

Finally, advocacy groups play a pivotal role in driving glaucoma awareness at both community and national levels. These organizations work tirelessly to promote legislative changes that improve access to eye care services and funding for research.

By supporting these groups, individuals can contribute to broader efforts aimed at preventing vision loss due to glaucoma. Staying engaged with advocacy initiatives not only enhances personal knowledge but also empowers individuals to take an active role in promoting eye health within their communities.

Support Groups and Community Programs

Support groups and community programs play a vital role in the prevention and management of glaucoma. Individuals diagnosed with glaucoma often experience a range of emotions, including anxiety and uncertainty about their future. Engaging with support groups provides a safe space for patients to share their experiences, learn from one another, and gain insights into coping strategies. T

hese groups can foster a sense of community, helping members feel less isolated and more empowered in their journey toward eye health.

Community programs focused on eye health offer valuable resources for individuals concerned about glaucoma. Many local health organizations and non-profits conduct educational workshops, free eye screenings, and informational sessions about glaucoma prevention. These programs aim to raise awareness about the importance of regular eye exams and early detection, which are crucial in preventing vision loss associated with glaucoma.

By participating in such initiatives, individuals can enhance their understanding of risk factors and the significance of proactive eye care.

Moreover, support groups often provide access to expert speakers, including ophthalmologists and optometrists, who can address specific concerns related to glaucoma. These professionals can offer tailored advice on managing the condition, including medication adherence, lifestyle modifications, and the latest advancements in treatment options.

Members can ask questions and receive guidance, which is invaluable for those navigating the complexities of their diagnosis. This direct line to expert knowledge helps demystify the condition and encourages informed decision-making.

Networking within support groups can also lead to the discovery of local resources and additional community programs. Participants often share information about nearby clinics offering specialized services, financial assistance for eye care, and transportation options for those who may have difficulty getting to appointments.

This exchange of information can significantly enhance the quality of care individuals receive and ensure they remain connected to the resources they need to manage their eye health effectively.

In conclusion, support groups and community programs are essential components in the fight against glaucoma. They not only provide emotional support but also serve as a platform for education and resource-sharing.

By connecting with others facing similar challenges and accessing community resources, individuals can take proactive steps toward preventing glaucoma and maintaining their eye health.

Emphasizing the importance of community engagement in eye care can lead to better outcomes and a more supportive environment for those concerned about glaucoma.

Continuing Education on Eye Health

Continuing education on eye health is vital for individuals concerned about glaucoma, as it empowers them with knowledge and resources to make informed decisions about their eye care. Glaucoma is often referred to as the "silent thief of sight" due to its gradual onset and potential for irreversible damage before symptoms become apparent.

By staying informed about the latest research, treatment options, and preventive measures, individuals can better protect their vision and overall eye health.

One key aspect of continuing education is understanding the risk factors associated with glaucoma. Factors such as age, family history, ethnicity, and certain medical conditions can increase the likelihood of developing this condition. Regularly reviewing these risk factors can help individuals identify their susceptibility and encourage them to engage in proactive monitoring and preventive strategies.

Educational resources, such as workshops, online courses, and webinars, can provide valuable insights into how these risk factors interplay and the importance of early detection.

Furthermore, advancements in technology and treatments for glaucoma are continually evolving. Staying updated on the latest developments in eye care technologies, such as advanced imaging techniques and new medications, can significantly impact an individual's management of their eye health.

Many organizations and eye care professionals offer seminars and informational sessions that focus on these innovations. By participating in these events, individuals can learn about new options for diagnosis and treatment, enabling them to discuss these advancements with their healthcare providers.

Additionally, the role of nutrition and lifestyle choices in eye health cannot be overlooked. Research has shown that a diet rich in antioxidants, omega-3 fatty acids, and other essential nutrients can contribute to better eye health and potentially lower the risk of glaucoma.

Continuing education should include information on dietary recommendations, exercise programs, and stress management techniques that support overall wellness. Engaging in community programs or online forums dedicated to healthy living can provide motivation and accountability for individuals looking to adopt healthier habits.

Finally, peer support and community engagement play a significant role in continuing education for eye health. Joining support groups or participating in local health fairs can foster connections with others facing similar challenges and provide a platform for sharing experiences and resources.

These interactions not only enhance knowledge but also encourage individuals to remain proactive about their eye health. By cultivating a community focused on education and support, individuals concerned about glaucoma can take meaningful steps toward preserving their vision and enhancing their quality of life.

How To Prevent Glaucoma

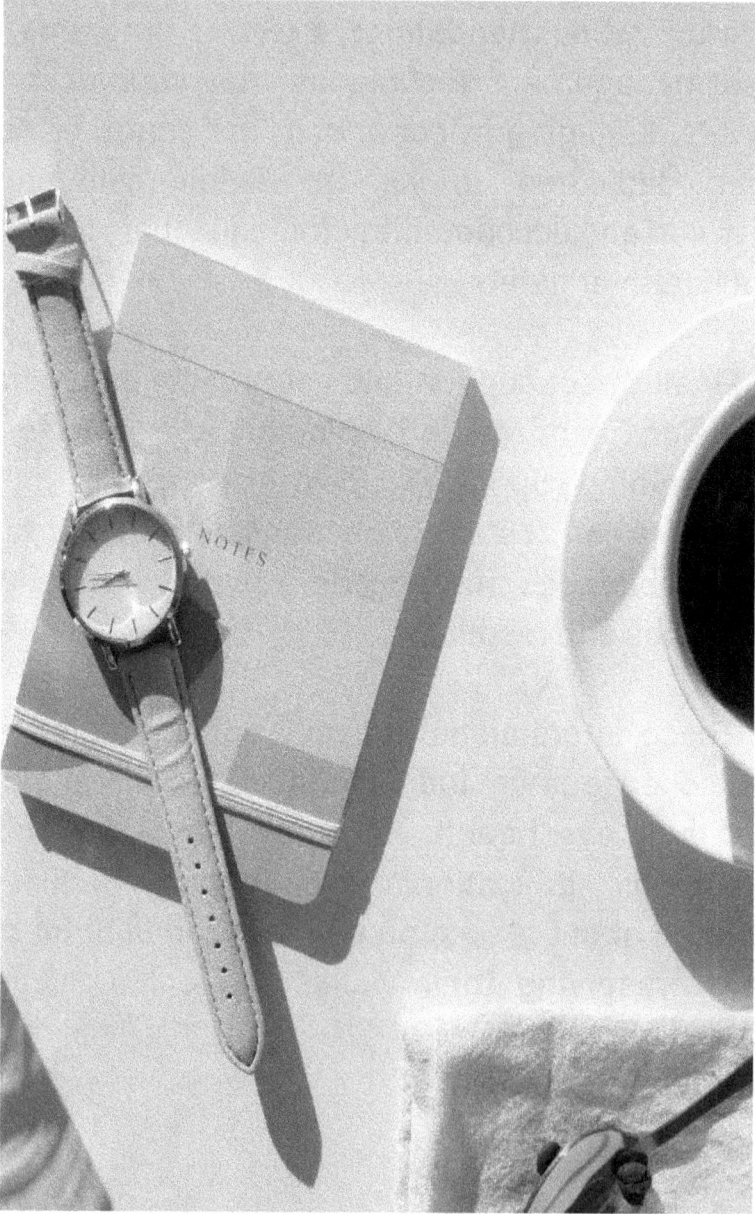

Your Action Plan for Healthy Eyes

Chapter 9

Creating Your Personal Action Plan

Setting Goals for Eye Health

Setting goals for eye health is a crucial step in preventing glaucoma and maintaining overall vision wellness. To begin, it is essential to understand the specific risks associated with glaucoma, such as age, family history, and certain medical conditions like diabetes.

By identifying these risk factors, individuals can establish personalized goals that address their unique situations. Setting clear, measurable, and achievable goals can motivate individuals to take proactive steps towards maintaining their eye health.

Regular eye examinations are fundamental to preventing glaucoma. Aiming for a comprehensive eye exam at least once every two years, or more frequently if recommended by a healthcare professional, should be a primary goal.

These visits allow for early detection of any changes in eye pressure or other indicators of glaucoma. Individuals should also track their family history of eye diseases, as this information can help healthcare providers tailor their recommendations and screenings.

In addition to regular check-ups, lifestyle modifications play a significant role in eye health. Setting goals related to diet and exercise can significantly impact overall well-being and, consequently, eye health. Incorporating a diet rich in fruits, vegetables, and omega-3 fatty acids can provide essential nutrients that support eye function.

Furthermore, establishing a routine that includes regular physical activity can help maintain healthy blood pressure and circulation, reducing the risk of glaucoma.

Another important aspect of goal setting is education about glaucoma and its prevention. Individuals should aim to educate themselves on the disease, its symptoms, and treatment options. Joining support groups, attending workshops, or reading reputable literature can enhance understanding and empower individuals to make informed decisions regarding their eye care.

Knowledge is a powerful tool in preventing glaucoma, as it fosters a proactive approach to eye health.

Lastly, individuals should set goals that involve open communication with their healthcare providers. Discussing any concerns or symptoms related to eye health can lead to more effective management and prevention strategies. Keeping a journal of any changes in vision, medications, and lifestyle factors can facilitate these conversations.

By actively participating in their eye care, individuals can create a comprehensive action plan focused on preventing glaucoma and ensuring lifelong eye health.

Tracking Progress and Adjustments

Tracking your progress in preventing glaucoma is essential for maintaining optimal eye health. Regular monitoring allows you to assess the effectiveness of the measures you are taking and make necessary adjustments to your action plan. Start by documenting your daily habits, including dietary choices, exercise routines, and adherence to prescribed medications.

Keeping a journal can help you identify patterns that may contribute to changes in your eye health, allowing for a more proactive approach in your prevention strategy.

Incorporating regular eye exams into your routine is another critical component of tracking progress. These assessments provide valuable information about the condition of your eyes, including intraocular pressure levels and the health of your optic nerve. Make sure to schedule comprehensive eye exams at least once a year, or more frequently if recommended by your eye care professional.

During these visits, ask questions about your eye health and the effectiveness of your current prevention strategies, as this feedback can guide necessary adjustments.

Another effective way to track your progress is by utilizing technology. Various apps and devices can help monitor eye health and remind you of appointments and medication schedules. Many of these tools also allow you to log symptoms and side effects, providing your healthcare provider with valuable data during consultations.

This information can be crucial in determining whether your current approach is effective or if modifications are needed to better align with your health goals.

Dietary and lifestyle adjustments play a significant role in preventing glaucoma. Keep an eye on your nutritional intake by tracking the consumption of foods rich in antioxidants, vitamins, and minerals beneficial for eye health. Consider incorporating more leafy greens, fatty fish, and nuts into your diet.

Additionally, monitor your physical activity levels, as regular exercise can help lower eye pressure and improve overall health. If you notice stagnation in your progress, reflect on these aspects and be open to altering your habits to better support your eye health.

Finally, it is important to remain adaptable and responsive to any changes in your eye health. If you observe any new symptoms or changes during your self-monitoring or eye exams, promptly discuss these with your eye care provider. Be prepared to adjust your action plan based on professional recommendations and personal findings. By actively engaging in tracking your progress and making necessary adjustments, you empower yourself in the prevention of glaucoma and the maintenance of healthy eyes.

Seeking Professional Guidance

Seeking professional guidance is a crucial step in preventing glaucoma, a condition that can lead to vision loss if not managed properly. Regular eye examinations by qualified eye care professionals are essential for early detection and intervention.

These experts, including ophthalmologists and optometrists, possess the training and tools necessary to assess your eye health comprehensively.

During an eye exam, they can measure intraocular pressure, check for optic nerve damage, and perform visual field tests, all of which are vital in identifying early signs of glaucoma.

Understanding the risk factors associated with glaucoma can help you communicate effectively with your healthcare provider. Age, family history, and certain medical conditions such as diabetes or high blood pressure can increase your likelihood of developing this eye disease.

Being prepared to discuss your personal and family medical histories during your appointment can equip your eye care professional with the information needed to tailor a preventive strategy specifically for you. This proactive approach not only aids in early detection but also allows for the implementation of preventative measures suited to your unique circumstances.

In addition to routine eye exams, seeking professional guidance may also involve exploring additional screenings or tests recommended by your eye care provider. For instance, if you have a higher risk for glaucoma, your doctor might suggest more frequent assessments or advanced imaging techniques to closely monitor your eye health. It is essential to follow through with these recommendations, as they can significantly improve the chances of catching any changes in your eye condition before they progress to more severe stages.

Education plays a pivotal role in glaucoma prevention, and eye care professionals can provide valuable insights into lifestyle modifications that may help reduce your risk. They can offer advice on maintaining a healthy diet rich in antioxidants, staying physically active, and managing stress effectively. Furthermore, they may recommend specific exercises or activities that promote good eye health.

By fostering a partnership with your eye care provider, you can create a comprehensive prevention plan that encompasses both medical and lifestyle factors.

Lastly, seeking professional guidance extends beyond just initial consultations. Continuous communication with your healthcare provider is vital as new research and treatment options emerge in the field of ophthalmology. Regularly attending follow-up appointments and staying informed about your eye health journey enables you to adapt your prevention strategies as needed.

Remember, prevention is an ongoing process, and collaborating with professionals in the field will empower you to take charge of your eye health and significantly reduce your risk of glaucoma.

How To Prevent Glaucoma

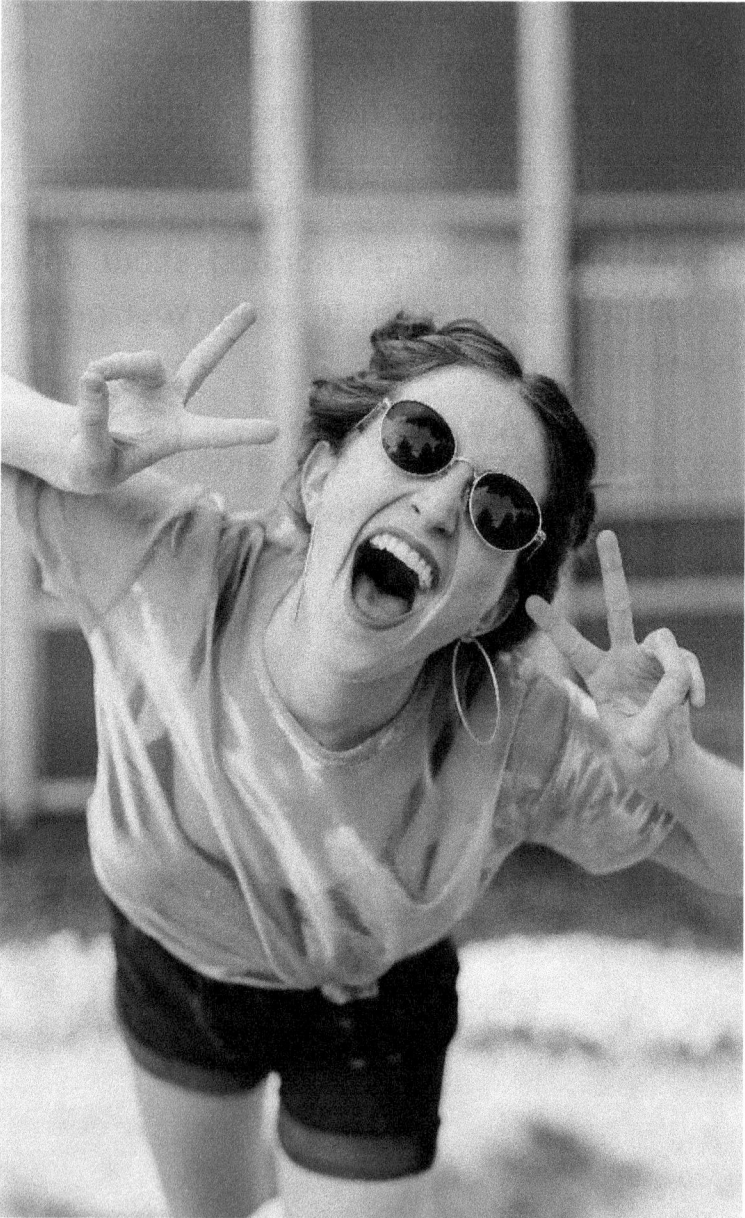

Chapter 10

Conclusion and Next Steps

Recap of Key Points

In the journey of understanding glaucoma and its prevention, it is essential to revisit the key points that have been discussed throughout this book. Glaucoma is often referred to as the "silent thief of sight" because it can progress without noticeable symptoms until significant damage has occurred.

Recognizing this, it is crucial for individuals to be proactive in monitoring their eye health and seeking regular eye examinations. Early detection plays a vital role in managing intraocular pressure and preventing irreversible vision loss.

One of the primary factors contributing to glaucoma is elevated intraocular pressure (IOP). Regular eye exams can help identify individuals at risk by measuring their IOP.

It is advisable to have comprehensive eye assessments, especially for those with a family history of glaucoma or other risk factors, such as age, ethnicity, and certain medical conditions like diabetes. Understanding these risk factors empowers individuals to take preventive measures and engage in discussions with their eye care professionals about their specific risks.

Lifestyle modifications are another critical aspect of glaucoma prevention. Engaging in regular physical activity, maintaining a healthy weight, and eating a balanced diet rich in fruits and vegetables can support overall eye health.

Additionally, managing systemic health conditions, such as hypertension and diabetes, is essential, as these conditions can exacerbate the risk of developing glaucoma. Stress management techniques, including mindfulness and relaxation exercises, can also contribute to maintaining optimal eye health and lowering IOP.

Adherence to prescribed treatments is crucial for those diagnosed with glaucoma. For individuals already undergoing treatment, understanding the importance of consistent medication usage cannot be overstated. This includes eye drops and any other prescribed therapies designed to lower IOP.

Education on the correct application of medications, as well as the implications of missing doses, is vital in preventing progression of the disease. Open communication with healthcare providers can lead to adjustments in treatment plans that better suit individual lifestyles and needs.

Finally, staying informed about the latest research and advancements in glaucoma prevention and treatment can empower individuals to take charge of their eye health. Participating in community awareness programs, support groups, and educational workshops can enhance understanding and foster a collective effort in combating this disease. By remaining vigilant and proactive, individuals can significantly reduce their risk of glaucoma and protect their vision for the future.

Encouraging a Proactive Approach

Encouraging a proactive approach to eye health, particularly concerning glaucoma, is crucial for individuals who are at risk or already concerned about this condition. Proactivity in eye care involves more than just attending routine check-ups; it encompasses a comprehensive understanding of one's risk factors, maintaining a healthy lifestyle, and actively participating in preventive measures.

By taking charge of their eye health, individuals can significantly reduce their chances of developing glaucoma or mitigate its effects if they have already been diagnosed.

One of the most effective ways to adopt a proactive approach is through regular eye examinations. Eye exams are essential for detecting glaucoma in its early stages, often before symptoms become apparent. Individuals should schedule comprehensive eye exams at least once every two years, or more frequently if they have risk factors such as a family history of glaucoma, age over 40, or other medical conditions like diabetes.

These exams typically include tests that measure intraocular pressure and assess the optic nerve, which are vital for early diagnosis and management of glaucoma.

In addition to regular check-ups, understanding personal risk factors is critical. Individuals should educate themselves about their family history, ethnic background, and lifestyle choices that may contribute to eye health. For instance, African Americans are at higher risk for glaucoma, and those with a family history should be particularly vigilant.

Moreover, lifestyle factors such as diet, exercise, and smoking can influence eye health. A balanced diet rich in antioxidants, regular physical activity, and avoiding smoking can all play significant roles in preventing glaucoma.

Furthermore, individuals should be aware of the symptoms associated with glaucoma, even though many people may not experience noticeable symptoms until the condition has progressed. Knowing the warning signs, such as peripheral vision loss, can prompt individuals to seek medical attention sooner.

Additionally, staying informed about the latest research and advancements in glaucoma treatment can empower individuals to engage in conversations with their healthcare providers, ensuring they receive the most effective care and management strategies available.

Finally, fostering a supportive community around eye health can significantly enhance individual motivation to adopt a proactive approach. Joining support groups or online forums dedicated to eye health and glaucoma can provide valuable resources and encouragement.

Sharing experiences and strategies with others facing similar concerns can create a sense of shared responsibility, making it easier for individuals to stay committed to their eye health. By building a network of support and information, individuals can be better equipped to take charge of their vision and actively prevent glaucoma.

Final Thoughts on Eye Health and Glaucoma Prevention

Understanding eye health is crucial for everyone, especially for those concerned about glaucoma. This condition, which can lead to irreversible vision loss, often develops without noticeable symptoms until significant damage has occurred.

Therefore, awareness and proactive measures are essential in preventing glaucoma and maintaining overall eye health. Regular eye examinations are the cornerstone of prevention, enabling early detection and timely intervention. By prioritizing eye health through routine check-ups, individuals can significantly reduce their risk of developing glaucoma.

Education plays a vital role in glaucoma prevention. Many people are unaware of the factors that increase their susceptibility to this disease, such as age, family history, and certain medical conditions like diabetes and high blood pressure. By understanding these risk factors, individuals can take informed steps toward mitigating their risks.

Awareness campaigns and educational resources can empower individuals to seek regular eye exams and discuss their family history with healthcare professionals, leading to earlier detection and better management of eye health.

Lifestyle choices also significantly impact eye health. A balanced diet rich in antioxidants, vitamins, and minerals can contribute to maintaining healthy eyes. Foods such as leafy greens, fish high in omega-3 fatty acids, and colorful fruits and vegetables can bolster eye health and reduce inflammation.

Additionally, regular physical activity not only benefits overall well-being but also helps manage systemic conditions that can exacerbate glaucoma risk. By adopting a healthy lifestyle, individuals can take proactive steps in their glaucoma prevention efforts.

The role of medication and treatment cannot be overlooked in the discussion of glaucoma prevention. For those diagnosed with elevated intraocular pressure or early signs of glaucoma, adhering to prescribed treatments is critical.

Medications, whether in the form of eye drops or oral medications, can help manage pressure and prevent progression of the disease. Furthermore, staying informed about new treatments and advancements in glaucoma care can offer additional options for those at risk. Engaging with healthcare providers about the best strategies for individual situations is essential for maintaining eye health.

In conclusion, a multifaceted approach is necessary for effective glaucoma prevention. Combining regular eye exams, education on risk factors, healthy lifestyle choices, and adherence to treatment creates a comprehensive action plan for maintaining eye health.

Individuals concerned about glaucoma must take an active role in their eye care, fostering a proactive mindset that prioritizes prevention. By doing so, they can safeguard their vision and enhance their quality of life, ensuring that they remain informed and empowered in the face of this potentially debilitating condition.

Author Notes & Acknowledgments

First and foremost, I would like to express my deepest gratitude to the people who inspired and supported me throughout the journey of writing this book. This project would not have been possible without their unwavering belief in me and their invaluable contributions.

To my wife, thank you for your constant encouragement and understanding. Your love and support have been my anchor during the challenging times of researching and writing this book. Your belief in my ability to make a difference in people's lives has been my driving force.

I would also like to disclose that this book contains some renewed artificial intelligence-generated content. I really appreciate very recent technological innovation by outstanding scientists and of course our reader's understanding.

Lastly, I want to express my deepest gratitude to the readers of this book. I sincerely hope the strategies and methods outlined within these pages will provide you with the knowledge and tools needed to truly make your life much better. Your commitment to seeking any good solutions and willingness to explore multiple methods is commendable.

Author Bio

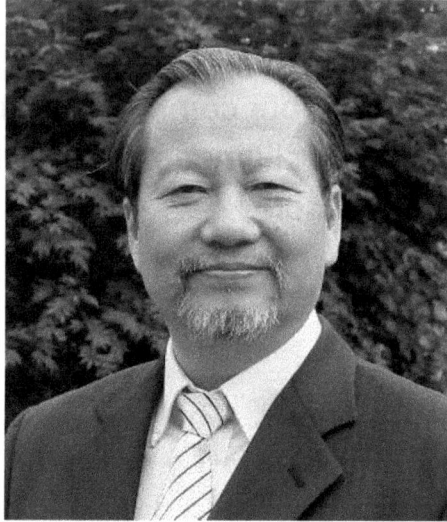

Johnson Wu earned his MD in 1982. With over 40 years of clinical experience, he has worked in hospitals in Zhejiang and Shanghai, China, as well as the Royal Marsden Hospital (part of Imperial College) in London, UK. Upon the recommendation of Sir Aaron Klug, the president of The Royal Society and a Nobel Prize winner in Chemistry, Dr. Wu was honorably awarded a British Royal Society Fellowship. He has published over 100 medical books in many countries and currently practices medicine in Canada

www.ingramcontent.com/pod-product-compliance
Lightning Source LLC
Chambersburg PA
CBHW060248030426
42335CB00014B/1632